Weight Loss Mentor

Making your weight loss a fun empowering experience you will be proud of.

By Marina Aleksandra

This book is not a scientific work.
It's based entirely on my personal experience,
thoughts and research.
There were a number of books I read
throughout my life that led to this spiritual
adventure and could give you more of the
technical, in depth information about
certain aspects of this weight loss
program. I will make a list of those books
at the end and I highly recommend them.
We all know the saying "everything is for a reason".
Well, I believe, gaining weight is for a reason as well.
As human beings we have to go through
a number of eye opening experiences
in life to learn to appreciate
what we have.

Acknowledgments

I want to thank my friends and family for being the way they are and teaching me the lessons of life that gave me power and strength to realize what's truly important.

I also want to thank the World for taking good care of me and giving me all those precious gifts along the way I won't ever forget.

Thank you!

Contents

Chapter 1

Introduction

It's been true for centuries that falling in love is one of the easiest ways to lose weight. You lose your appetite, sleep, thirst and without thinking twice about it or doing anything special you become a better you - with a better body and mind. And if it could be as easy as it sounds this would be the ultimate weight loss program.

Unfortunately in the real world with millions of options around and all the obstacles along the way, it's becoming more and more complicated to open up that true feeling within yourself or to find the person you could love. Well, here is where you can start. Start by loving yourself. Make it simple and learn everything you can from this difficult relationship.

Weight loss program introduced in this book requires a lot of commitment and positivity, but it will teach you to be patient, to protect, to have courage and to never give up. I call it: "one month weight loss program". Throughout this book it's referred to as "one month" or "this month", not because that's how long it'll take you to lose all the weight you want, but because that's how long it'll take you to give yourself a taste of what you could be like, that's how long it'll take you to realize how spoiled and unorganized you are, how much work you personally need to do to become that ideal you. You could reach your weight loss goal in two weeks or in a number of months. All depends on how much you need to lose and how closely you can follow the system.

It's not a secret that if you want to change anything or anyone around you, you need to start by changing yourself: by evaluating your own perceptions, your own desires and abilities, by finding what's important to you and what you're willing to do to reach that ultimate goal.

One month is such an unnoticeable period of time in the eyes of a lifetime, but in the eyes of the present one month could be the lifetime itself, during which you could make great changes within yourself and accomplish unbelievable results.

First thing you need to start working on is the feeling of rejection. Our minds are designed in the way of multiple comparisons, influenced by the judgements from previous experiences. Tell you what! Don't judge, don't compare, don't reject it because it's simple! It works. This system will be constantly changing your attitude and lifestyle from lazy "couch potato" to the engaged person willing to help all those around, willing to show them that there is a way - a way of commitment to live your life!

I'm a firm believer that you should love yourself the way you are without involving God in it! Don't say God made me this way, he gave me those extra pounds and low energy! God did not intend for you to be fat and lazy. We do it to ourselves. So since you made yourself this way: either be happy with your creation and stop complaining or get a hold of yourself and become the master of your body and mind!

For those of you who choose to fight, please note that this is a friendly fire sort of war. You are your own enemy, and it's not about killing the enemy! It's about changing the perception and views of our beings, so you could polish it into something beautiful, full of love to yourself and others. Full of happy, changed and peaceful thoughts that come out of hard and patient work. Today You are God. You are creating what you Love and can be proud of!

Food for thought:

Rejection. It's a negative response, denial or refusal. The original meaning of this word is "to throw" and it is exactly what this feeling does, it throws you off from the right track.

Falling in Love. This term is used to describe a feeling of love that is very strong and passionate but not necessarily permanent. Feeling of love arises when your six senses agree on one thing: you like what you see, you like what you hear, you like what you taste, you like what you touch, you like what you smell and you like the sensation in your body. When your brain agrees on all six - you fall in love.

Comparison. It's an estimate of similarity and differences triggered by our senses and experience.

Judgment. It's a formation of opinion based on previous conditions and experience.

Experience. Experience is a perception of knowledge that comes from observing and participation.

Laziness. Laziness is a lack of desire to be active physically or intellectually.

Overweight. To determine if you're overweight, ask yourself if it causes health problems. Causes of being overweight could be overeating, oversleeping, lack of exercise, emotional imbalance, low self-esteem, insecurity, poor digestion and many more. Drugs used for weight loss could weaken digestion and make your case worse by ruining the process of nutrition absorption. When the body doesn't receive the nutrition needed it sends a message to the brain that it's hungry no matter how many times you eat, making the eating process into a bad habit.

Perception. Individual opinion about a subject or an object influenced by your senses, memory and experience.

Present. Only very few people live in the present, most of us are just getting ready to live later. Present is a moment that you can not stop or capture, you can only live it or lose it, enjoy it or suffer in it - the decision is up to you. And don't forget that somewhere between yesterday and tomorrow is hidden that best time to accomplish anything in your life.

State of mind. Happiness as well as freedom is a state of mind. You are only as free and happy as your mind lets you be. If you're in charge of your mind you can control your future and bring happiness to your present.

Chapter 2

Commitment and Attitude

I talk a lot about commitment, it scares me how many times I say this word. But... - there is no other way. Only if you're fully committed to trying this for one full month - you will be able to accomplish great results. If you try it for a day or two and then quit, I can't help you, no one can! Go buy some miracle pills and stick with that.

I like my body, I adore it! Not just on the outside but on the inside as well. I know how much 24/7 work it does for me. We breathe 24/7, our liver, kidneys, stomach and all the other things we don't even know the names of take care of us day in and day out without any rest whatsoever!!! And what do we do in return? How ungrateful are we? We don't work out, pop pills left and right, drink caffeine products like it's water, we're inside all day long and complain about how hard and empty our lives are!

Even if you got noone in this world you got responsibility to all those little parts of your being that do such an honest job for you keeping you alive. Your responsibility is to take good care of them, to let them rest, give them right foods, not starve and overwork them with poisons.

Think of it. You are lazy, but your body is overworked. The loads of work are so high it gets stressed out and depressed. Just like you when you don't have a day off for even a couple of weeks at a time. Now imagine working for a number of years without a minute of a break!

The greatest part about it, that your body doesn't mind. It wants to work for you! It wants you to live and be happy! It rewards you when you're good to it. Feeling of peacefulness, natural high, it gives you adrenaline when you need extreme. It's ready to spice up your life at any given moment with all the sensations your body has to offer.

It makes you laugh and cry, when you are both happy or sad to ease the pain or deliver more joy. Now this is commitment!!! Can you do a fraction of it? Can you do for your body a fraction of what your body is doing for you?! Can you take responsibility for your actions and stop blaming everything and everyone else!? If yes, continue to read. This book is for you.

Now we need the right attitude. Remember the feeling of being in love? I truly hope that all of you at one point or the other of your life felt this beautiful, uplifting feeling. It is better to have loved and lost than to have never loved at all. Only this feeling can show you the attitude I want you to have - of "can do anything for as long as it takes without wanting much in return,"- just be close to the one you love, just be next to that one, just watch the one you love sleep.

Full of love, full of compassion, full of energy and positive thoughts! You are the observer. Don't get mad at yourself - no anger, don't judge yourself - it's all just a perception. Just observe... Observe your body, what it does for you. Know that you're doing something good for it for a change. You're not going to ruin it with harsh diets or dehydration, or working out till you faint...

No! No! And no! No miracle pills either. Do you even know what's in those pills or do you care?! Not really, ah? So why would you throw all those things in your body, like it's some kind of a garbage can? No diet teas that rip your guts out. None of that! Just take care of yourself for a change and watch nature work. Simply observe and be positive.

Food for thought:

Commitment. It's a firm agreement that could be quite challenging, especially if it's an agreement with yourself.

Attitude. Manner of carrying oneself, that could influence an individual to adopt or reject specific behavior.

24/7 work. An average heart beats around a hundred thousand times a day, it acts as a prime mover for the circulation of the blood. With each beat it moves a certain volume of the blood over and over and over. And it's safe to say that when your heart quits its job and stops - you die...

Breathing is another matter of life and death. In a lifetime it performs four hundred million or so operational cycles. It occurs spontaneously and without conscious attention or supervision. It is the only in and out process of your body that you can control with your conscious mind: making it slower or faster, deeper or more shallow. In Buddhist philosophy it is believed to be the bridge to reaching enlightenment and understanding your soul.

There is a constant life and death process in your body, where the old cells die and get disposed of, and the new cells are born and continue the Life. It's called the "Circle of Life". Even though this process is completely unconscious, your consciousness does play a big role in what kind of new cells are born continuously in your body. The food and nutrition choices you make, the water you drink, the air you breathe are creating and nourishing that new Life.

Mind. It's believed in Buddhist philosophy, that a person whose mind is undisciplined remains in the constant state of suffering.

Risks of Being Overweight. High blood pressure, high cholesterol and high triglycerides, heart disease and stroke could be the end to this journey of obesity. It also contributes to angina and sudden death by heart disease or stroke without any signs or symptoms. Diabetes, another cause of early death, heart disease, kidney disease, stroke and blindness. Several types of cancer are associated with being overweight. Sleep apnea, that can cause a person to stop breathing for a short period of time during sleep and heavy snoring; in the long run it can cause daytime sleepiness and even a heart failure.

Osteoarthritis - joint disorder that often affects your knees, hips and lower back. Gallbladder disease and gallstones are more common in overweight people, rapid weight loss can actually increase the chance of developing it.

Observer. One that observes without participation. When I say observer in this book, I mean it the yogi way. It is believed that our soul is a quiet observer of the world. The best way to observe is by being equanimous, without using the human nature of emotions, judgment and comparison.

<h1 align="center">Chapter 3</h1>

<h1 align="center">Don'ts</h1>

Things I don't want you to do:

1. Don't be negative. Like I said earlier you need to get rid of feelings of rejection, comparison or failure. It will not help, it will only raise doubts and excuses, it will slow the progress down or convince you to stop. I rather you not do it at all, than sit all day and send out all that negative energy of doubts in the air of this gorgeous Universe. Don't pollute it with your negativity, you're not the only one out here! We don't want your "presents" of rejection - enjoy and keep them to yourself!

We're all conscious beings. Nobody is making you do anything you don't want! Read it. If you don't like it - don't do it! ...and think of it as a money contribution for the cause.

2. Don't go to your friends and relatives and say: "In 30 days I will be 30 pounds lighter! I'm losing weight!"

Trust my personal experience, you do not want to put that kind of pressure on your shoulders! Perception, perception, perception... Too many questions you can't answer, too many doubts you can't defend against. Even though people are naturally good, public opinions are not. And your mind will already have a lot to deal with. Don't rush it! Don't stress it out! They will notice soon enough and by that time you won't even care about their opinion, you will know better.

During this month my personal suggestion is to say as little as possible. Save your energy, don't spend it on empty debates and arguments. You have a tough commitment and a challenging run in front of you. Don't worry, you'll tell them all about it later, when you're confident enough with your New Lovely Self!

3. Don't break your commitment. This first month is going to be the hardest. Not physically, but mentally. Remember, you're lazy and we need to break it. You're addicted to the off time, to the couch time or TV time. This is going to be the biggest challenge of your life! You will wake up in the morning and the "Junior" You will say: "No, not today! Let's do it some other time. I'm tired, I'm upset, I'm broke, I'm hungry..." But are you? Remember what's important and remember that this is temporary. Only one month, then you'll figure it out! You'll make your own decisions, your own schedule, your own lifestyle - easier to keep up with.

4. Don't miss your workouts. Now this is the first of two things that has to be scheduled in the beginning. In the beginning (the first two weeks or so) you need to work out every day at the same time plus minus one hour. This way your body will get easily accustomed to it. Sure if you've missed it for any reason and you've got some time later - do it later. But try your best to keep up with this rule. Make it a habit!

5. Don't drink a gallon of water when you work out. It's a challenge enough for your body to burn fat and calories for you to make it work even harder by processing water or anything else you might put in it. When you get thirsty, wash your mouth with water and spit it out. Your taste buds will send a signal to your brain that the water is in. If you're really thirsty, have 1-2 swallows, not more than that. You have plenty of time to drink water during the day as much as you want before or after...

6. Don't run - walk. Walking is one of the best exercises for your body. Human body is not made for running, we are one of the slowest runners of the animal kingdom. Walking on the other hand, as well as running, works on all the parts of your body in and out, only there isn't as much pressure on your heart and joints. It's easy and we all know how to do it! So do just that - walk!

7. **Don't eat if not hungry.** Hunger - this is an interesting concept. After this month you will notice how often we eat just for the hell of eating or because we're bored, or because it looks good. But ask yourself: "Am I hungry? Is my body hungry? What did I do to deserve this food today? Did I work out physically or mentally?" Don't lie to yourself! If your reply is: "Yeah, I could eat" or "Maybe I should eat something" ... The answer is - NO, you're not hungry! When your body is hungry there is no maybe, it will let you know. The feeling will be so strong you will have to stop and eat.

8. **Don't eat dead food.** Don't eat anything that looks or smells like it died last year. Market is flooded with foods like that! Remember those insides that work for you 24/7? Be nice, take care of them. Less you eat, the more you'll be driven towards healthy, nutritious foods. Let nature take you by the hand. But again, if you're really craving something and it's right there, even though you know it's not healthy, go ahead and have it. The whole theory is not intended for you to get stressed out because you can't have something. Use your best judgment! If you really want something - have it, make an exception.

9. **Don't eat after 6pm.** This is the second of two things that has to be scheduled. This rule is meant to be broken. Sometimes there was no other way, or there was no time, or it's 6:50pm and you've just missed it by 50 minutes... I have to say though if you're serious about losing weight quickly this rule works wonders no matter what and how many times you eat. The "6 o'clock" rule only seems easy. It's quite challenging! It makes your day go by very slowly after six until you go to bed. It divides your day in two. First part you eat, the second - you don't. It's better to eat right at six even if you're not hungry to keep this rule in tact.

10. **Don't get mad at yourself.** There is no point in getting angry. You're doing this for yourself and if you've missed a day of workout or ate after six, oh well, it's life and you're your own baby. Be patient! You're going in the right direction.

So what if it'll take one day longer!? In the next chapter I'll show you the combination of everything you need to do step by step. You don't have to follow all of them. Pick and choose. It's better than rejecting! You're the boss of your own life, you're the only one responsible for it. This workout system does work awesome in combination, but it's up to you. You don't have to lose all your weight in one month, sometimes it might just be better to take it slow.

11. Don't drink sodas or caffeine products. This rule is meant to be broken as well. But for the best results exclude all the sodas (they confuse your stomach about the amount of food needed to get full) and exclude all the products with caffeine (it over-stimulates your heart and colon). Like it was said before your body already works way too hard for you. Don't be that boss everyone wants to fire!

12. Don't look at the mirror. This one month mirror is going to be your worst enemy. It's like a public opinion except for you're judging yourself. Perception, perception, perception. I would rather for you to look inside, concentrate on your feelings, sensations, bring up your positivity and creativity. Think - that's what that big computer you have on the shoulders is for! Don't judge or compare yourself in the mirror with anyone else. Sure it's impossible not to look in the mirror for a month! But try to glance over versus stare, judge, compare and give verdicts to yourself.

13. Don't weigh yourself every 5 minutes. I understand the curiosity of: "How many pounds did I lose?"- but hold on to that thought. As well as the mirror this is your second enemy. Don't be a number. If you're going to weigh yourself, do it no more than once every two weeks. The concept of pounds will disappear from your head in no matter of time, you won't think in numbers anymore. What will matter is how you feel or how your clothes fit or how easy you move. Body weight is complicated and depends on various factors. Two of the most influential ones are muscle weight and water weight.

Approximately 80% of your body is water and there are a lot of diets out there that are based on dehydrating your body in order to accomplish weight loss. Well, you also accomplish bad health and rapid weight gain after you stop that diet. I want you to drink lots and lots of water! Pure water everyday. That's why if you weigh yourself very often you will not see the real results. All you will see is the reflection of how much water you have consumed that day.

The second factor is muscle weight and is even more complicated. Since you are working out your muscles start to get toned and become stronger, bigger and as a result - heavier. Therefore your muscles will gain weight while your fat cells get eaten away. The tricky part is that muscle weighs more than fat. So instead of losing weight you might actually be gaining it in the beginning. Just be patient and you'll get the results. Not only will you see them but you will feel them as well!

14. Don't get tired. Because you start doing so many more things a day your day will seem like four in one. You will have so much more time you haven't noticed before. First day is when you work out: you wake up, get ready, do something, go to the gym, work out, come back - all that will take 3 to 4 hours.

Second day is your normal day. You do what you normally do: you eat, drink, enjoy yourself, work, make money. This day is till dinner time at 6pm.

Third day is when you don't eat: it's after six, you're trying to stay relaxed, positive, and it's the longest part of your day! Most of the time even if you eat at 6 or 6:30 unless you go to sleep at 9 it's going to be pretty challenging. Don't mind it! It's all in your mind, you know you had dinner. If you're like me and like to have some drinks before going to sleep, watch out for the munchies.

And the fourth day is your sleep.

So, yeah! Once you start getting confused with how much you can do in one day, You "Junior" will slowly start telling you that you're tired. It's all in your head: you get all the sleep needed for your body, you get all the nutrition needed, you're not starving yourself and your workout is extremely easy. Don't listen to "Junior" and keep up the good work!

15. Don't overwork yourself. Some people believe you have to work out hard in order to lose weight. Please - not this month! Don't break yourself! Later, after this month, when you don't have to commit to one full month of gym without days off, you can add some new techniques and make your workout more challenging. But not right now!

It'll be hard enough to get yourself up in the morning without adding muscle pains and strains to it. Move the challenges toward the second, third month or so far... You've got your whole life in front of you! Do it when you only have to work out 2-3 times a week. Be nice to yourself. Love your body!

16. Don't drink pills. This one is very case sensitive. If you have to take pills for some serious condition it does not apply to you. This rule is only for an average healthy person that takes Advil or lots of vitamins or sleeping pills. Try not to put in your body any strange objects it has to fight or flush out later.

Headaches or sleep disorder - it's all temporary. Once you get yourself on the right track and your activity level will go up all these minor problems will fade away. All you need to worry about it keeping your spirits up high! And if that itself doesn't help, have a glass of red wine or even better - first warm it up for 30 seconds in the microwave and then drink it.   Hot glass of water with honey and lemon, and if you wish some green tea in it will soothe and relax you and is a great finish to any day. No more headache, no more sleeping problems, no more minor aches, no more stress...

Food for thought:

Failure. Failure should be seen as an early attempt to success, even though the original definition of "nonoccurrence of the expected outcome" is way more depressing. There are a lot of great quotes about it: "There is no failure except is no longer trying."- Elbert Hubbard; "Failure is a detour, not a dead-end street." - Zig Ziglar; "The season of failure is the best time for sowing the seeds of success."- Paramahansa Yogananda.

Doubts and Excuses. Doubt is a lack of certainty, a state of neither believing or disbelieving, that leads you to be undecided or skeptical about a subject without a particular reason. Excuse is an explanation offered in the hope of being forgiven or understood, used to serve as a justification of an act or an absence of an act, and to free from an obligation or a duty.

Public Opinion. Pulled judgment of the public in regard to a specific issue, influenced in majority by emotion and not facts or common sense. Statements of public opinion need to be treated with caution and only agreed with after careful research.

Mirror. There are two ways of spreading the light: to be the candle or the mirror that reflects it. - Edith Wharton.

Body Weight. Water accounts for nearly 80% of body weight. Day-to-day fluctuations in weight can often be related to water consumption, retention or loss. Weight gain can usually be explained by the increase of body fat, even though it can also be an increase in muscle weight, especially after illness or injury or during a new tougher exercise regime. In any case if you intake more calories than you spend, the overage gets converted into fat and stored in your body. In the case when it's the other way around, it's mostly fat that gets used up.

Walking. Don't walk in front of me, I may not follow; don't walk behind me, I may not lead; walk beside me and just be my friend. - Albert Camus.

The benefits of walking could be anywhere from cardiovascular health to helping alleviate depression. If you don't exercise much or at all talking to your doctor about your intention to walk is a good idea no matter what age you are. You don't have to be a member of a fitness club to get the benefits of walking, just go ahead and do it. Walking reduces the risk of heart disease, depression, lower back pain, risk of infection, increases muscular strength assisting in maintaining weight loss and increase in amount of "good" cholesterol.

In many cases you can burn more calories from a moderate walk than spending time on an exercise machine.

Sitting. Sitting slows down metabolism and may contribute to obesity, heart diseases, diabetes and metabolic syndrome.

Red wine. Small amounts of wine aid digestion and circulation, relax nerves and promote menstruation. The studies have found increased health benefits for red wine over white wine, including cancer protection and cardiovascular protection. Chemicals liable for those benefits are produced naturally by grape skins in response to yeast during fermentation. Wine is an alcoholic beverage, it's made from fermentation of the grape juice, and it can ferment without adding of sugars, acids, enzymes or other nutrients.

Beer. Diuretic. Can cause kidney stones. It's believed that in the long term it causes obesity, which could be argued that the real reasons are overeating and the lack of muscle tone. Moderate consumption decreases risk of cardiac disease and stroke. Long term effects could lead to development of alcoholism, alcoholic liver disease, and some forms of cancer. Brewer's yeast is rich in nutrients, that's why beer can contain magnesium, selenium, potassium or B-vitamins. Filtered beer can lose much of its nutrition.

Chapter 4

Step by Step Guide

Here is a sample of one full day I did for 2 weeks (after 2 weeks if you feel strong enough not to drop out you can modify the times of your workouts, if not - keep it up in the same regime):

5.30am - 6.30am Get up. Stay positive and calm.

6.30am   Out to the gym.

7.00am - 9.00am Workout:

1) Walk 3.5 mph (miles per hour) for 3 miles. To start - put the incline on 3, every half a mile bring the incline down by 0.5. After the second mile bring the incline down at the 2.3 mile mark and 2.6 mile mark. You should hit 0 incline at 2.6 mark. At 2.8 slow your speed to 3 mph, check your heart rate. At 2.95 bring it down to 2.5 mph. At 3 - you're done.

Remember to breathe. Take deep breaths, try to make them even. You're supplying your body with oxygen and getting rid of toxins at the same time. Your body works better and is more patient if you have rhythmic, even, deep breathing.

This whole exercise will take you approximately 55 minutes.

Note! Try not to talk in the gym. It's distracting, you will lose the big picture and might become a victim of public opinion. Concentrate on your body, you owe it that much!

Don't read when you do this exercise. It puts a lot of pressure on your eyes and might give you a headache, besides multiple eye problems.

Don't hold onto the handles, don't make it too easy for yourself.

When you get off the treadmill, hold on to the handles, you haven't realized it yet, but it's quite a workout, you've been walking with the same speed for an hour, you might get lightheaded for a minute or two.

Don't forget the towel and a change of clothes, because everything you walked in is going to be drenched in sweat.

2) Go to Sauna for 15 minutes. It doesn't have to be exactly 15, if you can't handle it, do less. Don't do more. It's tough on your brain and heart. This is to open your pores even more and flush more of the toxins out. It's great for your skin. Take a shower right after, before you go to the swimming pool.

3) Swimming pool. Swimming is one of the best, oldest and safest exercises. The best part is that you don't have to be professional at it, don't let those other guys intimidate you! You're here for a reason, just do your thing. I do 5 laps working my legs only, and 5 laps working only my hands. This will be explained in the later chapter. And ladies, you need to skip this part as well as Jacuzzi during that special time of the month.

4) Hot Tub - 5 minutes. Not more. It's better to go to the pool one more time than sit in a Hot Tub longer. If you overdo it, you will not want to come back. Besides this is more for contrast. It's good in small portions.

5) Shower. And your workout for the day is done!

9.00am Crazy cocktail. Normally when I get home I take my cocktail of nutrition. It's nothing complicated, but most of the people are not used to the taste of those items. You can choose not to do it, invent your own morning nutrition cocktail or do it separately throughout a day. The only thing I want to ask you is only take something if you know exactly what's in it.

  I take: a) 1000mg vitamin C
      b) 2 oz Apple Cider Vinegar
      c) 5-8 oz of Aloe Juice
      d) 2 oz of Pomegranate juice extract
      e) Distilled Water.

After this I can have another full glass of distilled water. The Nutrition section will explain more in detail about each one of these items and more suggested nutrients.

9.00am - 5.30pm You're on your own. Remember to eat only if you're hungry and for the best results drink only water, you can add some aloe juice to it or apple cider vinegar, honey or any other non powder nutrition you'll decide to work with. Use your imagination!

You can also drink organic milk products or juices not from concentrate. But remember that anything but water is just like consuming a meal, it has calories and nutrition your body has to work on, just like the food it has to be processed and you need to be hungry to consume it.

Sometimes if I want, I let myself have a cup of coffee or even an energy drink. It's not a boot-camp. It's life! Just be conscious about it! Remember that it's not good for you, and with time you will see how you stay away from those products more and more.

6.00pm Dinner time. Sure it can be plus or minus an hour, depending on your schedule. Six is an orienteer. Think of 6pm but "play it by ear." Don't stress out about it! Make your own rules.

7.00pm - 12.00am Again, you're on your own! Try not to drink anything but water in this section of the day. Being kind of a drinker, I let myself have some red wine, distilled water and club soda or sparkling water. I'm not saying that it's good or bad, but it works for me. So use your best judgment, make your own rules and watch out for munchies. After two weeks you'll get used to this schedule and it'll be a "piece of cake"!

  Twice a day without any special timing I do certain positive mindset exercises. I found that they work for me, make me feel better, make everything seem easier and more realistic to accomplish. There is more information about it in chapter nine.

  And last but not least is a once a week fast. This is to stabilize your built in "work with nature" mechanism.

  It's very simple and has been recommended and practiced for centuries. All you do is skip one full day of eating. Drink as much water as you want, preferably distilled (it doesn't have any added minerals and it's completely purified, it's great for flushing toxins and cleaning your organs).

  Just pick a day - Wednesday, Monday, Sunday - and stick with it!

  Today you have dinner, preferably at six and hopefully you don't drink too much; tomorrow you're only allowed water, it's easier if you're busy all day and don't have time to feel sorry for yourself' and day after, once you're done with your workout (you can make it a lighter one this day) have some breakfast, preferably starting with salad as your first meal.

Like I said earlier, it is quite simple, but it will challenge your mentality and beliefs to their core. You will need all the patience and commitment you can find within yourself to be able to stay on top of fasting and in control of your mind. The first advice about fasting is not to think about food and what you're doing, keep your mind busy elsewhere. The only bad news - controlling yourself doesn't get any easier during the first months... It will take time... More tips in chapter twelve.

Chapter 5

Life is Timeless

The concept of time is very complicated. It was created by humans. Not the Universe or God, not animals, but humans. It's almost like we enjoy counting down to our grave. Think about most of the sicknesses or bad things that happen to us, we blame it on time. On the mirage created by us so we have something to blame, so we don't have to take responsibility for our actions.

How many times have you heard:"Oh, it was just bad timing!" or "Time is cruel. It ages people!". Well, about that - time had nothing to do with it! You did it! You age yourself by what you do, what you eat, what you drink and what you think. I'm not saying that I won't age, but at least I know that it's all my decision making, it's nobody else's fault. I choose to drink, eat some french fries, take NyQuil, drink caffeine products, smoke and so far... I make those decisions knowingly and I do it to make my life easier or more fun. Whatever the reason is, it's nobody's fault, but mine!

Thinking is another interesting thing. We have the ability to convince ourselves in almost anything, no matter how outrageous it is! Here is one more phrase I like:"Time is of the essence." Of the essence for whom? Neither Universe nor God have the concept of time. They're timeless. They are Life and They are Timeless. They were there way before us and They will be there after.

Nothing in this life ever stops and starts counting its days, but us. Do we enjoy torturing ourselves with the boundaries of time?! Life only exists in the present and the present has no time, it's just it - present! You either enjoy it or screw it up by negative thoughts of the past or future, or by being impatient and thinking about the boundaries of time.

Note here I said "by negative thoughts"... Because there are a lot of moments in the past that are very pleasant and by bringing those memories back you actually increase the joy of the moment.

As well as the future: by thinking of the pleasure you're going to have or by dreaming of something beautiful you give yourself a sensation of happiness in the present and that's what life is all about - Happiness!

Next time you're waiting for something or someone, pay close attention to how this concept of time is making your life more and more miserable, how it's eating up your life, ruining your present. Catch yourself when you say: "How much longer, I've been here for 20 minutes! Damn, those minutes go by so slow. I wish it would be 5 o'clock and I would be home. This is like torture. Five more minutes and I'm leaving! Screw this!"

By this time you're getting angry, but why and at what? Learn to enjoy your life! Know that Life is Timeless and it depends on you how you spend it. Do you constantly think of what will happen next, what you're going to do next? Or you just slow down and enjoy it, knowing that any moment you lose in the present without doing something for you, without making yourself feel better, educating yourself, entertaining yourself or enjoying the beauty of life is a lost present, it's a wasted gift of Life. And if you can't enjoy this gift - you don't deserve it!

It sounds a little selfish, but it's not meant to be: we are doing something for ourselves every time we are doing something for our children and a lot of us enjoy and get pleasure from helping others, educating and entertaining those around us.

Next time you're stuck somewhere, think about it. Learn to enjoy your life. Learn to open your eyes and see what's going on in and around you. Think of the Universe. How endless it is. How it keeps movement in its chaotic, patient way. How much energy it has that you can tap into. How much power it's willing to share. How it doesn't grow old and just grows.

We don't need to know everything or find out everything in this one lifetime. What we do owe to ourselves and the Creator is to enjoy our lives to the fullest without harming the world within and around us.

The only thing that matters is - the present. Therefore, don't waste it! Be conscious. Life is a moment and that moment is NOW.

Luckyly for us there are a lot of those moments. So if something didn't work the way it should've, forget it and forgive yourself! There are plenty of chances to get it right. And if something should happen in the future you know about, a bad meeting or conversation you're not looking forward to, don't sweat it. Don't ruin your present! You'll deal with it when it's there. It's better to have that one bad moment than thousands of bad moments just thinking about it and playing it over and over in your head!

Remember! In the matter of the Universe our problems and miseries are not problems at all, they don't exist. There is a simple solution to all of them, it's called - Moving on... Life never stands still, but it is Timeless at the same time. Remembering this you might realize that the chaos of our lives is just an imitation of the movement of Life. Luckily our souls can stop and observe, making it easier to realize the beauty and the power of the Truth, called Life.

Food for thought:

Time. Time is eternal even though we pass by. Try not to say never, never is a very long time!!! Time is a treasure that you can't keep, you have to spend it. There is a constant war going on between us and this concept in which we are simply killing each other. The sad part is that, as human beings, we know a lot of ways of killing time and none of resurrecting it.

Eternity. Nothing is eternal but eternity. An average person that doesn't know what to do with this life, dreams about another one that would last forever.

Happiness. Repetition is the key to realizing and remembering: happiness is a state of mind. You won't get happy by getting a golden palace or the best car. You will get temporarily satisfied, but not happy.

There is no end to human cravings or desires. If you let it rule your life, your life will become miserable, and you will suffer in the endless attempt to acquire material things. To be happy you need to train your mind to be free of cravings and rejections, and try to stay balanced on the inside and out in any situation you might experience by observing reality as it is and you within it.

Universe. An ancient Buddhist scripture said: "In each atom of the realms of the universe, there exist vast oceans of world systems."

Chapter 6

Just Walk!

The whole "Life is Timeless" concept will help you a lot while you walk for an hour a day. You will probably catch yourself thinking a lot of the thoughts from the past chapter. So hold on to your patience and keep repeating to yourself: "Life is Timeless". See how your attitude will improve slowly throughout the month, how you'll be getting more patient, more able to enjoy your present.

Walking is a great exercise and since we live in a chaotic world we don't have enough of it. We mostly sit. We sit while driving, while working, watching TV or a movie, having dinner, conversing with a friend. No wonder we taught our bodies to be lazy! Right of teenage time, as soon as we get the car, we begin our sitting life. And only prolonged walking exercises could break that habit, slowly but surely giving you more confidence and energy. Making you more mobile, more alert and ready for the challenges of life!

I already said earlier why you shouldn't run, well, here is one more tip. You have to start slowly, and running is quite a workout! I have nothing against it! It's just not for everybody and definitely not for someone who hasn't worked out in a while! Your body will react with the objection to this sort of punishment and you might not come back to the gym after only a couple of workouts.

I want you to be patient and just walk, let your body get used to it and start liking this new activity before you do any changes. Just give it one month and then, when you're on your own and able to make clear decisions, do anything you feel like, anything you desire and think is good for you.

The main things to remember about walking:

1. **The Speed.** The speed you walk with is very case sensitive. I wouldn't dare to tell you: "You have to walk 3.5 miles per hour". Everyone is different. For some people 3.5 mph is running, for the others - it's too slow, they won't even break a sweat.

   Here is how I did it: I brought the machine up to the speed that I walk so fast that it's easier to run (which was 3.8 mph) and then dropped it down a little to a comfortable fast walking speed, where I can control my breath and the movement of my legs (which ended up being 3.5 mph). Once you find that speed on the first day - stick with it! Some days it'll be easier, some days it'll be harder. Just keep in mind it's only for one month, then - you'll make some adjustments.

2. **Milage.** I want you to trust me on this one and just do 3 miles a day. Not more, not less. Less is just not enough, and more will take way more time plus you'll get bored and tired in a week, you'll feel like it's a waste of time and drop out. Once you're done walking for a day there shouldn't be any feeling of tiredness; just a feeling of accomplishment and it's great if you feel like you could walk way more.

3. **Incline.** The reason I put an incline on is to trick my body into thinking that the more it walks the easier it gets. That's why I start with an incline on 3 and then every half of a mile I drop it down by 0.5. It works wonders! The first mile is always the hardest, the second one is easier and the third one is a "piece of cake". Not to ignore that the first mile on the higher incline you will drop way more sweat than on the second and the third.

4. **Breathing.** Try as much as possible to make your breathing equal. For example four steps inhale and four steps exhale. If you screw it up don't worry about it, just return to it later, don't get mad at yourself, no negative energy should come out of you. The main pressure should be on the exhale, that's when you lose weight and get rid of toxins, with the exhales.

Plus you don't need much help inhaling... So if they have to be loud make them loud. Big no-no! Don't breathe with your mouth. If you can't breathe with your nose, you're walking too fast. In and out, always with your nostrils. Close your mouth and leave it alone. It's not its job!

A lot of times when you try to pay attention to your breath your mind will wander away and you'll forget all about it. Don't freak out and start hating yourself - it's normal. Our brain is designed in the way that it likes to multitask, and it likes a good challenge.

Breathing is such a normal task for your brain it doesn't understand why you want it to watch your breath, that's when it gets arrogant and starts doing 2-3 things at once. Thinking about the present, future and past, jumping from one thing to another, being its normal self. Now you as a wise parent can't get mad and yell at your little "child", but slowly and gently bring it back to the task you want it to do.

5. **Thinking.** Even though I want you to watch your breath, I know that it's highly improbable doing it for an hour straight. So when your mind wanders away try to bring it to one of these subjects:

    a) <u>Thinking about your body.</u> What kind of work your body is doing for you at this moment. Watch and observe all the muscles that are currently working, feel how they move, try to constantly help them with your support and acknowledgement of their movement. Not physically, psychologically.

    Move your legs, feel your hands, shoulders, stomach when you inhale or exhale. Realize how much work your organs do for you on the day-to-day basis. Understand the responsibility you have to them, how much you owe them and what you're willing to do for them.

b) <u>Thinking about the time concept.</u> Every day when I walk I have to remind my lazy self about the Timeless Life. Our brain is so used to being pointlessly entertained by someone else's experiences it doesn't feel like being in the present in this particular body, stuck, walking. It's way rather watch a TV novel or News or listen about someone else's tragedies, so it doesn't have to think about itself, be responsible, make decisions and take proper actions. And you can't blame it!

This comes from years of brainwashing and being told what to do by our parents, TV, ads, your boss, or even God. Well, why would you want to start doing something right now? It means more work, you would actually have to think for a living. And even this book... Aren't you reading it because something or someone suggested you should?

Every time you catch yourself feeling sorry for yourself remember that Life is Timeless, so you're not losing any time, relax and enjoy the present as it is. As an inner "You" observe this moment, your behavior, educate your brain about your new philosophy, make your mind stronger by being patient. Get to know yourself on the whole different level and start falling in love with the new You.

c) If you catch your mind wandering away, <u>don't allow any negative thoughts</u>. No matter what you did, no matter how far your mind went or for how long - don't get upset or frustrated. You can't change nature, you can only educate yourself about it.

While you work out and throughout this month don't allow any negative thoughts. If you catch it - get rid of it, throw it out of the window, don't let it ruin your life, your present! It's not worth it. Keep your mind focused on the big picture. Don't make more negative energy than already exists in this world.

With every breath - breathe in the power of the Universe, the energy of life and breathe out your dreams and hopes - deliver the message back into space.

By doing this you let the Universe know what to work on. What's important and dear to you. What you want. It's listening to all your hopes and desires, to all your plans and it has all that energy to help you! Breathe it in - take its help, be patient, wait for the signs, and when it offers you a gift - take it and be grateful!

Likewise, when you think negative thoughts, - the Universe gets confused. It thinks that if you put so much thought into it, so much time and energy, if you're taking your time thinking about these ugly things, you probably really want it! You want bad - it gives you bad! It doesn't judge or discriminate against you. You just get what you ask for...

Every thought, every word is a signal for the Universe. Good or bad! All it does is say: "Your wish is my command!"

Learn to stay away from negative thoughts and more Positive will be happening in your life! Learn to control your life with the power of infinite love and great compassion for yourself and then others. Once you forgive yourself it'll be so much easier to forgive others.

At the same time when someone is throwing their negative energy in or around you: don't mind them, don't take their "presents" and get angry back. Simply breathe in deeply, even that negative air, and with the powerful help of the Universe breathe out complete positivity. Their mood shouldn't bother you, because the Universe and God is on your side. They will give you all the power you need to break down the ice into a soothing healing spring water.

6. Finishing up your walking cycle. Once you're on the 2.8 mark if your incline is not at zero yet, bring it completely down and this is the point where you need to slow your speed down and slowly bring yourself to a complete stop. Just like it's not recommended to make a quick stop after running, the same comes for walking fast. Be smart about it and listen to your body.

7. In general. Don't make a common mistake of holding the handles while you walk. The name of the exercise is walking, not Carrying Yourself. Let your hands be, just hanging there. They'll get plenty of workout when you swim or exercise in the water.

Walking without holding on to handles is very important for your posture, spine, breathing apparatus, stomach and leg muscles. Don't be lazy! It's better to slow your speed a bit than hold on to something.

There are two exceptions:

a) When you use a towel - always hold on or you might lose your balance;
b) When you're done and about to get off the machine - hold on, because you might get lightheaded.

Even though this whole chapter is about a treadmill machine and walking on it. If you don't have a gym membership or treadmill machine and you decide to walk in the park everything still applies to you.

It's just going to be a little harder. You need to find a 3 mile route or find out how many circles you have to do around the park. You need to keep a track of it and walk fast without slowing down or stopping.

You could also time your walk, this way you don't have to count the miles anymore: time how long it takes you to walk 3 miles, then set up your alarmwatch and walk.

8. Change of clothes. If you didn't sweat - you didn't work out! Either you were walking too slow or you weren't breathing or the incline is too low for you. Use your best judgment and fix what needs to be fixed!

When you stop walking the top part of your shirt should feel like someone just dumped a bucket of water on you. Do not be embarrassed or look at some other people that are there to hang out and chat or make an impression. You're there to work out! It's not a convention center - it's a gym!

 I found that less eye contact you make in the gym - more people leave you alone and more work you get done quicker. Once you get your mind and body back on the right track and once you change into different clothes go ahead and do what you want, make friends, chit-chat or go home and enjoy friends and loved ones you already have - it's up to you! No one can tell you how to live your life, they can only tell you how they live theirs.

 All this was to say - don't forget a change of clothes! Always have two sets of clothes going to the gym (including sucks and underwear).

 One of the greatest benefits of walking for such a long time is that during that hour you will easily come up with solutions for various situations of Life, be it your life or the life of others. Good luck and start walking your life! Baby steps... Be patient... Baby steps...

Food for thought:

Incline. Challenges the cardiovascular system without requiring speed, recruits lower back muscles to keep your body erect and provides a stretch to the calves. Small incline is suggested for the people with knee pains.

Breathing. Breathing techniques enhance walking and turn it into a more challenging exercise. Breathing cycle should start in the belly, open up the rib cage and finish up with your shoulders extending a little back. The exhale will go in reverse.

  Proper amount of oxygen is needed to help break down food into nutrients, to rejuvenate cells in the body and for your brain to function properly. We get barely enough, our air is polluted and most of the time our breathing is shallow and doesn't allow us to use the full capacity of our lungs. Deep breathing exercises are very helpful in the attempt to provide the lack of that supply.

  Breathing through the nose is very important. Nose is equipped with hair filters to get rid of dust as well as temperature regulatory function, to cool down or warm up entering air.

Chapter 7

Sauna and Health

This chapter doesn't need a lot of explanation, I'm not going to get deep into it. If you're curious about the proof of why saunas are good for you - research it.

All I'm going to tell you is that this is one of the easiest ways to drop weight, clear your skin and get rid of toxins. This is one of the oldest and laziest workout techniques out there. Where you have to do absolutely nothing! Just get in and stay there for a certain period of time.

Sauna is not for everyone. Some people can't stand a minute there - neither should they. If you have any kind of major health issues, especially heart related, it's better if you consult the doctor or a fitness specialist if the use of sauna is safe for you.

Personally, I'm a big fan of dry saunas. On my workout days I do 15 minutes a day. Don't do more than that! During my lifetime I've done anywhere from 5 to 40 minutes and I found that 5 is too short of a time to do any good for you and anything over 15 minutes overheats your brain to the point of fainting, which you don't want.

My recommended time is 15 minutes, if you can't do that much do at least 10 and slowly bring it up. Don't make yourself be in there if you're anxious to get out. Baby steps...

A lot of people like to go to the sauna and do pushups and sit ups. It's all good, but don't try it this first month. It's only for physically very fit people. You get tired and work your body way faster and harder in hot temperature conditions. You need to last a month going there every day for 15 minutes! You might just want to take it easy...

Let nature take its course and work for you. Get in and relax. If you know how to meditate, try that. If not - try breathing and the thinking themes from the walking chapter.

Food for thought:

Sauna. Dangers of the sauna include heat prostration or even heat stroke. A quick switch to cold water could cause an increase of blood pressure, so it's better to change different environments slowly. Benefits of sauna include some relief for asthma patients, chronic bronchitis, rheumatic diseases. And in moderation it's not harmful to almost anyone.

Chapter 8

Swimming and Hot Tub

You don't have to be a professional athlete to swim. A lot of animals if you throw them in the water will start swimming instinctively. Talking about great exercise for your joints!

If you don't know how to swim, maybe it's time to learn and in the meanwhile join the water exercise group. They have a lot of great exercises that will give your body the same effect as swimming.

I assume you're not a professional swimmer or you wouldn't be interested in reading this book. Now... I want you to forget everything you know about real swimming and what we're going to do is just try to stay on top of the water with only moving your hands or only moving your legs. Please, no supporting gear. You're not tricking anybody but yourself!

Throughout these exercises watch your breath (breathe slowly), don't freak out and enjoy the moment. It's better to do less laps, but do it the right way, than more with the floats. Don't be lazy. Remember, even though it's pleasant - it's still a workout!

These are the three exercises I want you to do:

1. **Swim only with your hands.** Put your hands in front of you, lay down on your belly and swing both of your hands symmetrically towards your body sideways as in breaststroke or "frog" stroke swim style. Forget the legs, just keep them together. You're working on your hand muscles right now. If you feel like you're going under water you need to do it faster. Keep yourself up, floating, and keep your hands moving constantly, don't stop till you reach the "shore".

In front - to the sides - in front under water - and to the sides. Your palms should be open and looking towards your body while swinging them towards the sides of your body, fingers together. When you straighten your hands in front of you try to do it as quickly as possible to avoid going under.

Be calm, patient and think about your breath and hand muscles. Feel your hands working and listen to your body. If it tells you a better way to do it, take its advice. If you can't seem to do it on your belly, turn around and do it on your back.

If you do it right you will feel the resistance of the water being moved by your hands, you will feel your hands' muscles, your core and your body moving forward.

2. **Swim only with your legs.** Have you ever seen a dog swim? Do just that but with no hands, imagine that your hands are tied, you can't move them, they can't help you. This is a great workout for your legs and abs. You can put hands to the sides of your body, in front of you or right under your belly. Be very patient with this exercise as it's very tiring. Take enough breaks between laps.

    You can also do it on your back. In that case I found it more challenging if you either move your legs very fast or make "scissors" like movements with the minimal bending of your knees.

I do 5 laps of legs and 5 laps of hands with a break between every lap. And I do: hands - legs, hands - legs, hands - legs, hands - hands, legs - legs. Done!

3. **This is not an exercise.** But this is great for relaxation. Just lay down on your back and try to stop all your thoughts. It'll be easier in the beginning since fat has a tendency to float and muscle drowns. So with time you will have to spread your hands and legs (starfish like) as far to the sides as you can to keep floating. Watch your breathing and enjoy!

If you can't do any of those exercises on your belly, do it on your back. But then don't skip on the number: five each - means five each!

Hot Tub is just for contrast. Don't do more than 5 minutes. Get in, enjoy it and get out! It's very good to help with all the minor pains you might have after workout and it's great for toning and clearing your skin. The only minus is all the chlorine most of the gyms use to sanitize water. Five minutes is plenty! If you have a hot tub at home - do that instead.

Food for thought:

Swimming. This is a great liberating exercise that gives you a full body workout without much pressure on joints and bones, while relaxing your nerves. Drowning, exposure to chemicals like chlorine and infection are the biggest risks of swimming in the pool. So be cautious and don't swim if you have any cuts, transmitted diseases or are allergic to any of the chemicals used to clean the pool.

Chapter 9

Positive Mind Set

The key to successful weight loss is to keep a positive mind set, positive thoughts. There are several ways to train your mind to be continuously happy. Some of them are based on realization of the basic truths of nature and the other ones are accomplished by convincing yourself that you're happy.

We'll start by programming ourselves to be happy. The goal is to convince your brain that you have everything you need and every second of every minute you keep getting more and more good in your life; that all your dreams are on the way to accomplishment and the Universe with all its energy is working for you!

Pick a phrase. It has to be pretty general, it can be a saying, a goal or anything at all. Make sure it's very uplifting and makes you feel like You are on top of the Universe. Write down that phrase nine times in the morning and nine times at night time. Keep doing it all month long without changing the phrase. While you write it, think of what you're writing and agree with it. It has to become your second nature. Throughout the day, if you feel blue or down, repeat that phrase as many times as you need to convince yourself of what it says.

You can use one of the phrases I write or pick a new one, make sure it's very positive! I write: "I flow in the stream of well-being. My world will take care of me. God opens the way where there is no way."

Second step is to stop being afraid. There is nothing in this life worth being afraid of, all you do by being afraid is waste the precious moments of your life!

There is really not much to be scared of knowing that you're the Boss of your mind and God and the Universe are on your side. You choose how you spend moments of your life - you choose what you feel: happy, depressed, calm, excited, in love, hating - it's all up to you, not to the person those feelings are towards, it's up to you!

The third step is to realize the constantly changing nature of life. Everything rises and passes, feelings and sensations come and go. Nothing is permanent in this world: not you, not the buildings in front of you, not your boss, not your job, not the ocean, not the space as we know it. All we can do is keep moving in this chaotic world and try to get the best out of it.

The person you were when you got this book - that person no longer exists. You, that's reading this book right now, - is a new You. It's the You with the constantly changing mentality, it's the You that lives in the present, it's the happy You if you let it be.

That's why being positive is one of the best things you can learn in this life! Sometimes you could just stop for one second and it's enough to see the beauty of the present, to change your attitude, see the big picture and enjoy your life.

If you have to be addicted to something be addicted to positivity, happiness, health, feeling of love and peace! With the way it works - the more you think or educate yourself about these concepts, the more it's going to work for you, the more changes you'll see in your life. Life is what you make it!

I wish you get all the strength of the Universe you need to make your life beautiful, to make it real!

Food for thought:

Fear. Fear is an emotion that's caused by the expectation of a real or imaginary danger. It normally appears as an unpleasant sensation of tension towards an object or situation. Mark Twain said: "Courage is resistance to fear, mastery of fear, not absence of fear."

Impermanence. Buddhist way of looking at the nature of life as constantly changing, without a beginning or the end. You can see the proof of that philosophical belief in everyday life by simply observing it: your body and mind are constantly changing, the people and animals are never the same, the trees and nature keep evolving. There is eternal arising and dissolution of the matter around you. That's how it always was and that's how it'll be...

Reality. The totality of all things. Reality is a two sided coin, in which most of the time you can only see the side closer to you, the side that is facing you.

Chapter 10

When to Eat

What seems to be a very easy concept is misunderstood by millions of people. We eat when we're bored, we eat when we watch TV, when we're depressed and so forth... All that is besides 2-3 meals a day which are supposedly required: breakfast, lunch and dinner. Majority of those times you're not hungry, not even close to it!

Recognizing hunger is difficult nowadays since eating became a habit, something to do when there is nothing to do. In most cases it's not a necessity anymore, it's a pleasure. Pleasure that has its own liabilities! Some of those liabilities are: excess weight, digestive problems, laziness, low energy level; and all that comes from one of the deadly sins - gluttony. Like I said, it's an easy concept that's very misunderstood by the people of the present.

Think of it this way. A long time ago in the Stone Ages people didn't have refrigerators or preservatives to keep their food properly stored or to make it last. Every day was a new day! Every day you would have to go find food for yourself and your family. There were no three meals a day. If you're hungry you hunt, fish or find some fruits, veggies, nuts or berries. But you would have to physically do something in order to eat, your body had to deserve the food.

Present time civilized people could not survive in the predator's environment - we're too slow, too lazy and don't have the energy needed. You can say thanks for that to the preservatives, soda drinks, excess amount of caffeine drinks, dead food with no nutrition and overeating, as well as present advertising mania that's pointed at triggering your cravings so companies could sell more and make more money.

Your bad health is very profitable! Nobody's going to teach you differently, nobody wants to teach you "healthy"! You need to teach yourself, it's your responsibility!

If you're naive and still think that advertising works for you, you need to wake up and "smell the coffee". Look closely at the ads, read the fine print, listen to what it says, what it warns you about and what it promises. Not just hear - Listen!

Most of the food ads are driven by gluttony, greed and visuals. It shows you a beautiful picture of what the food is going to look like, your brain gives a signal to your stomach, your stomach releases the juices, and here you go - you're ready to eat, you get sudden craving for that particular item. It's basic psychology, that has nothing to do with the benefit to your health!

Let me simplify this for you. When you do this one month program slowly but surely you will change your mentality about food, nutrition and health. I want you to concentrate on two points.

The first one is - don't eat if you're not hungry. That means: no snacks, when you watch TV, no early breakfast unless you're hungry, no set meals. I need you to get yourself once or twice to the extreme feeling of hunger, remember the sensation in your body, remember what "hungry" feels like and from that point on - eat only if you get close to feeling the same sensation. Eat only if you're hungry!

You don't have to sacrifice yourself and stop planning your meals, but you do have to clearly understand that the feeling of hunger has nothing to do with the food you eat, at that point you will eat almost anything.   There is no such a thing as preference when you're hungry.

At the same time as you go on this one month journey you will notice a stronger drive toward healthier, raw, organic, nutritious foods. You'll get full quicker and feel it on your own example that "our eyes are way bigger than our stomachs".

Don't mind anything that's going on in your brain, let the battle begin! The battle for a stronger and healthier you - the battle that you can't lose!

The second thing to remember is - if you're serious about losing pounds don't eat after 6pm. Now again you are your own Boss, so if you haven't eaten all day and it's pushing six, and you're still not hungry - go ahead and eat something. Not a lot, just something. This way you can't talk yourself into eating later. As a responsible adult you will realize that the feeling of hunger at nine is a fake because you've eaten earlier. You can't be that hungry and you can wait until tomorrow. You can eat all you want tomorrow!

Be positive! Don't punish yourself for anything! If you're hungry - you eat. The reason people lose weight quicker if they don't add calories after six is because in the night time your body slows down, it doesn't break down food as quickly, you don't have as many activities, you're about to go to bed and sleep and your whole bodily mechanism is getting ready to do just that - slow down and relax, which leads to keeping most of the calories you insert in your body at that time. Give it some rest and let nature take care of you.

Food for thought:

Hunger. Hunger is a cry of your body for nutrition. No matter how much you eat, if you don't eat the right food you will always end up being hungry. On the other hand, if you give your body what it needs, the feeling of hunger will disappear and you will be rewarded with the energy and great figure at the end.

The only cure is to consume more organic, unrefined, raw products and stay away from anything with preservatives, coloring, natural or artificial flavorings or spices (unless it specifies what kind of spices and you know exactly what those are). It will take some time to reeducate yourself, but it's way worth the effort.

Thirst. Thirst is the same way. The only way to get rid of thirst is to drink water.
That's all your body wants! If you're thirsty it needs water. Don't fool yourself and give
it "rehydration drinks", the best way to rehydrate is to consume plain, clean water.

Chapter 11

Nutrition for your Body

Nutrition is not necessarily food. It's basically anything your body can take out of something and use it to make itself healthier, stronger and more energized.

Sure, a big part of our daily nutrition is hidden in food. But food could be two types - nutritious and poison. Poison doesn't mean you'll die from it the minute you eat it, but it will slowly kill you by accumulating in your body, draining its strength without adding anything in return.

Today's food is full of preservatives and hormones, it's over fried, over boiled or simply old. A lot of businesses out there are just trying to make a buck, they need that food to sell and make profit, that's where you come in...

Mind yourself, listen to your body, think about it, take care of yourself! You don't need that dead chicken nugget, that's been in the refrigerator for a half a year!

No, you need nutrition, you need to feed your brain, liver, blood, you have responsibility to do so, - you need organic, clean, healthy foods. Don't say "no" to it before you even try it! Don't say "it's expensive". What do you mean it's expensive?! And your health is not?! If you put a half of the money you spend on your insurance and medicine into real organic food you won't need that much medicine - it's called preventive medicine.

Prevent yourself and your body from getting sick, keep yourself out of the harm's way. My advice is - eat good, eat healthy and don't overeat.

The other types of nutrition are supplement extracts, real juices and so far. It is very case sensitive and you really should do a little research, look into your needs and decide what's best for you.

 I will give you some examples of what you could be taking in the morning or in general, but the decision is up to you. You can adopt it or ignore it, add something or throw something out.

 Pomegranate Juice Extract. Pomegranate contains polyphenols, ellagic acid and punicalagin. Polyphenols promote antioxidant health, which helps fight cell damaging free radicals that can lead to oxidative stress and the risk of premature aging of cells. Punicalagin has been identified as the active compound responsible for maintaining and promoting cardiovascular health. You can find organic preservative-free "Naturally Pomegranate" on-line and at your local stores.

 Aloe Vera Juice. Aloe is a "miracle" plant with moisturizing and healing properties. Aloe juice has a very specific taste you would have to get used to, but the rewards are great. Depending on the sensitivity of your digestive system, you can drink it as often as you like, but it's recommended to start with 4 oz per day. Large amounts of aloe juice without getting used to it could cause diarrhea.

 Clinical studies indicate that aloe has curative properties in various digestive conditions. It could be taken internally or used externally, for the treatment of bites, blistering, burns, dry skin, gum and mouth disease, constipation, hemorrhoids, insomnia, kidney ailments, sunburns, stomach disorders, ulcerated skin and wounds. You can also find this supplement at your local stores.

 Unfiltered Organic Apple Cider Vinegar with no preservatives. It contains cleansing and healing powers, kills germs, viruses, mold and bacteria and aids in losing weight.

Here are just some of the ailments it can be used against: headache, warts and calluses, corns, sunburns, cleansing the skin, sores, poison ivy, varicose veins, dry and itchy skin, hives, bites, acne, fungus, baldness, muscle soreness, aching joints, arrhythmia, digestion, kidney and bladder problems, arthritis, mucus, constipation etc.

The taste of Apple Cider Vinegar is very concentrated and it has a very strong smell. It's best for intake with water or you can use it as a salad dressing. You can find it in the oil and vinegar section of the grocery stores.

Honey. For nearly 3000 years honey has been used by humans to treat a variety of ailments. It could be used as an antiseptic, in treatment of diabetic ulcers, in reducing the damage done to colon in colitis, as a treatment for sore throats and coughs, it may reduce odors and swellings, not to mention the nutrients it contains for your body giving it energy and strength.

Yogurt. Just plain white organic yogurt. It's believed to promote good gum and gastrointestinal health, and has nutritional benefits beyond milk. If you have to have a dessert, train yourself to eat yogurt with honey. It's way healthier and more satisfying than over the counter deserts you might choose.

Lemon. Fresh squeezed lemon in the glass of water is believed to clean the liver. It also helps to stimulate your metabolism. It has antibacterial values, could be used in facial masks, and it is a natural deodorant.

Chapter 12

Once a Week

This is the part about fasting. I highly recommend it. Full fast on distilled water once a week. Don't add anything and don't take anything out.

Just water and you. Distilled water is known to clean your body out of toxins, out of all those poisons we get throughout the week from air, regular water or foods. You will literally hear your body say "thank you" every time you finish your one day full distilled water fast.

It's easy, it's a no brainer. All you need is to control yourself, control your cravings and habits. You have dinner at six the day prior. Don't eat anything the day of fast, I mean don't put anything in your mouth other than distilled water for one full day. Go to sleep and you can have breakfast the next day as soon as you wake up. During the fast you can drink as much water as you desire. Flush those toxic poisons out and keep in mind - your body is doing a great deal of work this day. It's not busy eating and breaking down the food, it's busy cleaning the mess you've been creating your entire life. Give it a break: don't work too hard, don't think too much!

I found it easier to do one of two things:

- Work that day to keep yourself busy without thinking much about not eating. If you eat with your coworkers, tell them you had a big breakfast or lunch and you're not hungry yet. Don't tell people what you're doing. Even if they want to support you, the nature of public opinions or "I'm better than him" or "I can break him, I think that would be funny" or "...just do it for me this one time" will succeed. It's better for you if you don't give it a chance! You know what you're doing and that should be good enough for you.

- Or have a day off. Take it easy that day, don't talk to anyone, don't go anywhere, if you feel like sleeping - sleep. Read, daydream, make plans for the future and this particular day I do not suggest thinking about the present.

Staying in the present with all the good intentions in your heart, realizing and knowing that you're doing an awesome cleaning procedure for your body will not help you this day! Cravings are much stronger than you might think! An average person never really thinks about it, but craving for something you can't have is stronger than your mind power.

Just deal with it, always staying positive, it's just one day - and this one day if you have to - live in the future, daydream, relax, no pressure, just good feelings, don't think about what you're doing, don't think about food or what you'll have for breakfast tomorrow, be ready to be very patient. It also helps if your refrigerator is empty that day or if you just don't open it at all, forget you have it!

One thing to remember about the day after fasting is that you need to do anything possible for your first meal to be vegetarian (easier on your stomach), healthy (organic salad would be great) and light (no potato, chips, mayo, corn, meat or pastry). None of the heavy to break down food. I usually have a salad with lemon juice and minimum condiments.

I need to mention a couple of exceptions for this chapter. If you can't stop smoking, drinking or taking pills for a full day I do not recommend water only fast, in those cases it's better to do 100% organic juice fast. It's the same principle as the water fast only you're also allowed the juice of your choice. Like I mentioned earlier it's better to modify than completely reject.

People that don't feel strong enough to do water only fast should start with the juice fast and slowly bring themselves towards the water one. Once you get used to the taste of aloe juice it could be one of the most ideal juices to use that day as it has zero calories and tons of healing powers.

Some weeks when it feels harder and you feel weaker, rather than not fasting at all do the aloe juice & water, lemon juice & water, honey & water, apple cider & water or any combination of the above mentioned items, do 24 hours instead of a full fast, but - don't give up!

Food for thought:

Fasting. Fasting makes it easier to bring your body back to the lifestyle full of good habits. It gives your body internal cleaning, aids in losing weight, gives you a clearer perspective of the world, and helps you become more pure physically and spiritually.

Distilled water. It's a main weapon used to flush the toxins and dead cells out of your body without adding any new ones. Distilled water is deeply purified, it's free of all substances, be it minerals, sodium or chemicals, it simply goes through your body and cleans it from the inside out.

Not eating. Remember: nothing gets rid of hunger better than thirst. In this hard battle between brain and your heart you must not let your stomach win.

Bad food. Think of it this way - thanks to refrigerators, now we can eat old food.

Patience. The first thing you lose when you start a diet is your patience.

Metabolism. Metabolism slows down during the night, this is the time your body uses to recuperate and re-energize itself after a long day.

Chapter 13

After Six

This one month or for as long as you keep it up this is going to be the longest part of your day. It's going to become the longest and the most challenging part of your life! It doesn't matter if you go to sleep at 6:05pm or you stay up until 3am. The mental message of NOT is stronger than any positive feelings or realizations. Once your brain gets the signal that it can not do something after a certain time it takes a great deal of patience, control and making it into a habit to stay on top of that rule!

Our brains refuse the NOT signal, they become revolutionary, they like their freedom of choice and don't like to obey. Breaking yourself is harder than breaking others. You are your own Boss. It's a huge responsibility, you've got no one to answer to but yourself. All the mess ups, all the failures - you've got no one to blame, but yourself.

And that's where it gets very tricky, because blaming yourself will not fix anything - it will slow the process down. In this case it'll slow down the process of getting healthier, getting up and getting on your feet. And since this is the least desirable outcome, we have to forgive ourselves for everything we did wrong or we might do wrong. There are plenty of chances to get it right. If you've missed one, grab on to the other one and continue on the path to the right track. When you're ready you'll get it right! Life is Timeless. And time is not of the essence!

After this one month or when you reach that ideal look for yourself, the six o'clock rule is the easiest way to maintain your figure. Even if you eat anything you want throughout a day, as many times as your body desires, you will not gain any weight for as long as you do it! You can also modify it to every other day, which is more realistic for a busy, fast paced lifestyle. If you do modify it I would suggest to keep exercising at least three-four times a week.

I understand that it sounds kind of over the top, like a lifetime commitment, but not to worry! It's not that bad! You will rarely have to think about it. By that time it won't seem like an issue. If you put your best effort in this one month program, your body will start craving exercise, it will get used to not eating after six, and it will make it easier for you to choose the right type of food.

And once again - if you do mess up and lose your way in the future you will always know what to do! You won't get depressed, you will just look at yourself like a child that did something wrong, forgive that child and start again, start it all over from the beginning. Baby steps... When you're ready - you WILL get it right!!! You've got all the time in the world to get it right.

Chapter 14

Control your Brain

It seems like the brain is in control of your body, but throughout this month, when you walk for an hour a day or when you don't eat after six, pay attention and observe how weak it really is. How jumpy and indecisive it really is! How it skips from one subject to another without finishing up the thought. How it runs away from painful subjects and can't keep an objective perspective on a problem.

Both your conscious and unconscious minds are like the South and North pole of the Earth. They're so similar, but are even greater different. They don't seem to even know about each other, and don't care what the other one is doing and why.

One - is an arrogant, egocentric teenager that needs constant control and supervision (conscious); and the other one - is over obsessive workaholic parent that has to have everything done by the book and on time, it reacts to every sensation in your body with an adequate reaction that you never even have to think about, it needs no supervision, it's always on time and it never rests (unconscious).

So what is the solution? How do we control these two completely different creatures within us? How do we make it work?

Every person needs to find that answer for themselves. There is no remedy or magic potion. You have to stop, look into yourself, observe all your thoughts, emotions, sensations, see who controls what. Make those two the best friends! Make them work together, study each other, understand each other. Live, play and learn!!!

Every time you remember about it, every time you can - try to stop your thoughts, look around yourself, stop moving for a minute. Hold that thought. And observe. Look into yourself, see how hard your body, heart, breath keeps working for you. Relax and don't move a single muscle.

Don't think. Don't compare. Don't judge! No positive or negative, just you. Simply observe... Only through observing yourself like that will you see the true nature of the soul. You will see how pure and patient it is, how unbiased it is, how calm and strong it really makes you. And it's all inside of you, you - are all you need to be happy and accomplished!

So control your brain, your emotions. Lead your soul into being happy and satisfied with the reality of the moment. Remember that even if the events of the present moment might seem unpleasant, they're there for a reason, they're there to teach you a lesson or to bring your soul to the whole new level.

Don't say "No" to your life, and take all the gifts and lessons it has to offer. Be thankful and celebrate it! Might as well! Especially if you believe in eternity...

Don't get stuck in the past. It's gone!!! If the memories are bad - let them go, forget it! Don't let it ruin your present!

Present is a new life with new possibilities and it's going to be what you make it. Sad, happy, angry, successful and so far... Past is just a memory, a reflection of life before the present.

Don't confuse your brain by taking the present and stuffing it into the past, it doesn't appreciate it, it stops working towards progress, towards new. It gets stuck, forgets all about the present or the life itself, and keeps living in the labyrinth of your memories not even bothering to look for the way out. No! It doesn't keep living - it simply exists...

If the memories are good - bring them back once in a while. I don't blame you! I've got some great memories stored in the "Past" folder of my brain. Memories that create sensation of happiness, success, feeling of love, compassion - those are always welcome! I hold them dear to my heart and every time I need an "afternoon pick me up", instead of drinking a cup of coffee, I have a couple of minutes of sensations from the past!

Since our brain hates and refuses reality, it's too jumpy for it, too impatient (now I don't want you to get too mixed up: soul is patient, brain is not), by observing, you will notice how it jumps from past to future, future to past and so far. If it has to jump somewhere at this particular minute let it be the future. Future is open to possibilities, it lets you explore new horizons, new ideas, make plans, dream, hope, and figure out the ways to enjoy your life even more.

According to Buddhist philosophy we suffer because of two main sensations: craving (when you desire something so much you feel you can't live without it) or aversion (refusal of the situation or object created in the present, past or future).

Both of these are the creatures of the present, they are the ones you need to be aware of and know how to fight them. Don't let them get the best of you and steal your present! Both of the feelings are created toward something you can't have, don't have or wouldn't have for quite a while. The exercise in the beginning does a very good job in fighting and realization of these issues that can make our present miserable.

I want you to also understand the difference between feelings and sensations. Feelings are something you feel on the psychological, spiritual level. It's not associated with your body, even though it's triggered by your senses or sensations, like falling in love for example: you see it, you hear it, you smell it, you taste it, you touch it and you get a pleasant vibration in your body; your brain comes up with a response or a judgment - you are in love. This is one of the most complicated examples where all your senses and sensations have to agree.

Feeling of greed is easier: you see something, and you decide (the judgment is) - that looks so good I have to have it!

Sensations on the other hand are the emotions of your body that are triggered by your five senses. When you see something and feel a weird vibration in your stomach - that's a sensation. So you could say that sensations are more of the physical vibrations of your body, either pleasant or not. Sometimes people even refer to it as "six sense", because it happens unconsciously, on a deeper level in our bodies which we have no control over.

Chapter 15

When and What Not to Drink

To achieve the best results during this month you need to stay away from all soda drinks (except sparkling water or Club Soda), all caffeine drinks, beer, all drinks made from concentrate, all supplement drinks (like vitamin waters with coloring) and not organic milk products.

This month you need to do everything possible to help your body clean itself and purify your thoughts as well as the perception of the world. Once you cut all these drinks out you'll be surprised how limited your options are, but... - they are so much more satisfying at the same time!

Water. The best is distilled water. Drink as much water as you desire throughout the day! Don't have too much water right before or after a meal, as it feels you up and gives you a feeling of fullness. It also dilutes the stomach fluid and makes it harder to digest food. And I'll remind you again - not to drink anything, even water, while you work out! You can drink anything you want half an hour prior or after working out. If you get extremely thirsty go ahead and have 1-2 sips of water or just swirl it in your mouth and spit it out.

Juice. Anything that says "made from concentrate" is not a juice. Please, if you care about your health, look at the label. You don't need all those fake fillers! Get only 100% not from concentrate, organic juices. You can have them any time except when you fast or work out. Beware of calories in juices! Drinking a glass of juice could be a full meal for your body.

Milk. Adults shouldn't have too much milk as it's designed to help your body grow. But if you have to have it, use only organic milk. Drink very little of it, just enough to kill the craving. Absolutely no milk products on fasting days, during workouts or after 6pm. Let your body rest as milk products are heavy to break down.

Coffee and caffeine based drinks. These are energizers. But don't get fooled by a thought of easy energy, like "it gives you wings". The "wings" it gives you are not free - caffeine drinks put lots of pressure on your heart, giving it a fake burst of energy that is very short and addictive. You think if you have another one the feeling will last, but it doesn't. It's never enough and before you know it you get the shakes from all the caffeine and sugar in your body. Your hands are shaky, you've got a headache and still no energy, you don't know what to do and feel left out. During this month you'll get your energy back, just give it a try, give it a little time.

Less energy or vitamin stimulants you'll drink - more energy you will get at the end! If you drink a lot of coffee or energy drinks the first week is going to be tough. Keep thinking positive and understand the harm you're doing to your body by using those. Be responsible, it's your body, take care of it and it will take care of you!

Sodas. Most sodas are full of calories, artificial sweeteners, preservatives, coloring and carry no nutrition for your body. It does no good and it stops the signals your body uses to tell you it's full. I'm against all soda drinks, the only thing they're good for, in my personal experience is a hangover.

There is one exception - club soda (which is just carbonated water) or sparkling water. Every time you have an urge for soda drinks ask for club soda. You can't drink a lot of it, and if you add a lime or lemon you're actually helping to clean your internal system. Another big plus is zero calories. Sure sometimes we get used to a taste and we feel craving for a particular item. Well, be mindful: have a sip instead of a glass and have a glass instead of six refills.

Alcohol. Beer, wine and liquor. I can't tell you to drink or not to drink. It's just like smoking: we all know the dangers of alcohol and cigarettes, but for one reason or another, after weighing pluses and minuses, some people choose to do it and some people choose not to. As long as you hold on to the other rules, if you don't overdo it, drinking will not be your biggest issue on the way to success. After knowing your limits, the hardest part about drinking during this month will be staying away from food after six and waking up in the morning.

So be patient with yourself, sometimes that drink is the exact item that will get you through and sometimes it's not. Analyze your habits, commit to the rules, make a list of exceptions and follow them.

Absolutely no drinking or smoking during the day of the fast! It's only one day - you can do it! Think about the rest of your body, how grateful it's going to be if you do this one thing for it. If you can't do a full day - do 24 hours! Baby steps... Be very, very sensitive to yourself and your cravings. It's better to do something, than nothing at all - just ignoring life and closing your eyes when you see a big picture, just looking away when you see an obstacle. You are a responsible, wise parent of yourself, sometimes you just have to find a different approach to get your message through.

Try also not to drink or smoke when you get out of fast, at least not till the second meal. With time your body will guide you, it will show you the way and make it easier to choose wisely. Life is timeless and you have all the time you need to become that ideal you.

Chapter 16

Forgive Yourself

No matter what you did, no matter how many rules you broke, how many days you've missed, how negative your mind might seem sometimes - do not get mad at yourself, do not get angry. Let it go and start all over, start where you left out.

What happened a day or five minutes ago doesn't matter! You are a new and improved You every minute of every day. You keep growing, experiencing and learning.

Don't be that angry boss that no one likes! Your body works very hard for you day after day, imagine if it would quit?! Your responsibility is to lead it on the path of life, by being in charge and making right decisions about its well-being. But if something messes up along the way - learn from it, understand it, research how you talked yourself into breaking a particular rule, what was your reasoning, how you used it and at what time. Analyze what happened and make adjustments to your attitude: "Oh! Now I know this trick! I won't let it work on me again!"

You have to forgive yourself for all the mess ups! First you're doing this for yourself - maybe you weren't ready at that moment or something caught you off guard. Second, if you get mad at yourself, human nature will win, and you will look for someone or something else to blame, which will set your progress back way further than any mistakes you might've made! You will stop believing in yourself and will think that the outside world has the actual power over you.

Your body itself is like a huge universe, where you are the creator. Well, that's a lot of responsibility, a lot of pressure. Don't give up and don't let that universe die!

Forgive yourself for everything in the past, and now, when you're on the right track, help yourself along the way, be positive, be patient. You've been getting yourself in this hole your whole life! It'll take some time to get out of it, but there is no doubt you're getting out!   Forgive yourself so you can learn to forgive others.

Food for thought:

Forgiveness. Mental process of ceasing to feel anger, resentment or other negative sensations toward the object that has done something to justify such response.

It is misfortunate how weak we are in fighting the sins, but we have no right to blame anything or anyone for it, as we might not ever fully understand the reason for their existence; give it the right time and causes any of us could've been an unwilling participant or accidental weapon of destruction toward yourself or others.

Chapter 17

Falling in Love with Yourself

I love to see myself slim down! There is something very satisfying in thinking: "Oh, I guess I can do it! And I was about to give up! Wow, I can't believe how easy it is! All I had to do was try!" I love my new attitude! I love the way I look at life and people! I love my new me!

...that easy! It's all inside of you! Happiness, freedom, power, success, love are all just the states of your mind! Today - you caught a fish - and you feel Successful, you have no money from it, but the feeling of success is there. Tomorrow - you'll be getting ready for work and you'll look at your eyes in the mirror and see how much deeper they are than you actually thought, and you will fall in love - Fall in Love with Yourself.

Then - you'll go outside and it's a beautiful day: not too cold, not too hot, with some clouds, just enough for your imagination to go wild, and you'll feel the wind that's like a breeze even though there is no ocean - you will suddenly feel Happy! And then - when you sit on some boring work meeting, you can't leave, you're stuck there for at least an hour, minutes are dragging, but you know that in the big picture of life this meeting means less than the pimple on cow's ass; so you're listening with one ear and let your mind go free, let it dream on, let it run wild and imaginative - and you will feel Free!

Think of the person you want to be, think of the qualities you want to have, in detail visualize that perfect image of You... Right now! This moment - feel it!... Who you are and what you are like? Visualize it and be it!... Everytime you lose your way, come back to this exercise, adjust your perception and become who you want to be!!! It won't always be easy to be happy or to be in a good mood, but as long as you try you have a chance to succeed.

    This should be enough reasoning for you to Fall in Love with Yourself. You ARE the reason for what you feel and how you feel it! And if you're in love with yourself I guarantee you'll be happily in love for as long as you live! You are going to be Your Happily Ever After...

    And again! You have to love yourself in order to know how to love others!

Chapter 18

Second Month and The Life After

As much as I would like to say that you'll lose all the weight you want in one month, I can't. It won't be true! Everyone is different. I don't even know if you want to lose 5 pounds or 255 pounds - the results WILL vary. But I could vouch for - you're on the right track.

You're working on your attitude, you're working on your perception, you're becoming a better, more understanding person. Don't worry! Stick to the program as close as you can and the pounds will melt.

Now, don't do more than one month straight of this system, it might wear you out. You need a break of at least a month. My personal recommendation for the second month (which will let you drop even more weight while toning and building your muscle mass) is:

Monday, Wednesday, Friday - stick to the same workout: one hour fast walk, you can add a little 5-10 minute run at the end if you feel like it, 15 minutes sauna, 10 laps swim (you can modify your swimming to your desires) and 5 minutes hot tub.

By this time your eating habits should be different. They should be more thoughtful. The only rule you need to hold on to is no eating after six. Be mindful of what you drink and eat. Remember, even though your month-course is over - your life is not, and life depends on how often and what you put in your stomach! If you can - hold on to the once a week fast. It'll do great things for you in the long run!

Tuesday, Thursday, Saturday - same eating habits. These are your off days. All you have to do in the comfort of your home is 100 pushups and 300 situps. Later you can adjust the numbers, but for right now do just that. Don't think too much about it! It souls like a lot, but I'm not there to supervise you - You are!

And I'm not telling you to do it all at once. No! Either you do 1 pushup 100 times throughout a day or 100 pushups at once is up to you. Neither I'm going to spend time explaining the techniques. It's easy - use any internet search engine and you will find hundreds of techniques online. Any of those will do! I don't care if you do it the military style or girly style, if you modify it or cut the corners. All you need to keep up with is a number! Gorgeous body - here You go!

Sunday - complete day off. But if you feel like doing something, find a yoga class, do it once a week to begin with, it will give you the flexibility you've never dreamed of, it will make your muscles ageless!

That's it. Now you're on your own. It's a big, beautiful world out there! Use it to your advantage, enjoy life and everything in it! Do your best to reach for the stars and the stars will reach for you. After a second month, after you evaluate yourself, you can choose to stop, continue or modify the program. The main point remains the same. You are your own Boss, so act like one!

I wish you all the luck in finding your way and fighting your demons! Good luck and may the power of the Universe be with you!

Widening the Circle of Love. His Holiness the Dalai Lama, translated and edited by Jeffrey Hopkins.

The Art of Happiness. A Handbook for Loving, His Holiness the Dalai Lama and Howard C. Cutler, M.D.

The Four Noble Truths. The Dalai Lama, translated by Geshe Thupten Jinpa, edited by Dominique Side.

The Miracle of Fasting. Frozen Throughout History For Physical, Mental and Spiritual Rejuvenation. Learn to Live in Agelessness With Bragg's Complete Life Extension Program. Paul C. Bragg, N.D., Ph.D. with Patricia Bragg, N.D., Ph.D.

Super Power Breathing for Super Energy High Health and Longevity. Paul C. Bragg, N.D., Ph.D. and Patricia Bragg, N.D., Ph.D.

Water The Shocking Truth That Can Save Your Life. Paul C. Bragg, N.D., Ph. D. and Patricia Bragg, N.D., Ph.D.

<u>Personalized schedule</u>

____

____

____

____

____

____

____

____

____

____

____

____

____

<u>Notes</u>

<u>Recipes</u>

www.ingramcontent.com/pod-product-compliance
Lightning Source LLC
Chambersburg PA
CBHW081808250726

48653CB00010B/3835